OZEMPIC

ONCE A WEEK WEIGHT LOSS INJECTION USES, STORAGE, INTERACTION AND MUCH MORE TO PRODUCE A DRAMATIC RESULT

LEO O. NORDISK

CONTENTS

INTRODUCTION

This book aims to provide a comprehensive guide on the proper use and storage of Ozempic, a medication used for the management of type 2 diabetes. Ozempic, also known as semaglutide, is a peptide receptor agonist-glucagon-like 1 (GLP-1). This is a once-weekly injectable medication that helps control blood sugar levels in people with type 2 diabetes.

OVERVIEW OF OZEMPIC

Ozempic works by mimicking the action of a hormone called GLP-1 in the body. GLP-1 is responsible for stimulating the release of insulin, reducing appetite and slowing digestion. By activating the GLP-1 receptor, Ozempic helps regulate blood sugar, leading to better glycemic control.

Unlike other GLP-1 receptor agonists, Ozempic has a longer duration of action. This means that a single injection can provide continuous blood sugar control for up to a week. This prolonged action makes it convenient for people who prefer a once-a-week treatment option.

Ozempic has been shown to be effective in reducing fasting and post-meal blood sugar levels. It has also demonstrated additional benefits, such as promoting weight loss and reducing the risk of cardiovascular events in people with type 2 diabetes. These additional benefits make Ozempic a valuable tool in overall management of diabetes.

IMPORTANCE OF PROPER USE AND STORAGE

The correct use and storage of Ozempic is essential to ensure its effectiveness and maintain patient safety.

Proper use involves understanding the prescribed dosage, injection technique, and following the recommended schedule. On the other hand, proper storage practices are necessary to maintain drug stability and avoid degradation.

By following proper Ozempic usage guidelines, people with type 2 diabetes can optimize their treatment results and minimize the risk of complications. Consistent and precise administration of the medication allows for better blood sugar control, thereby reducing both short-term symptoms and long-term complications associated with diabetes.

Apart from using Ozempic correctly, it is equally important to store the medicine properly. Improper storage can compromise the potency and stability of the medication, making it less effective or even harmful.

Temperature, humidity and exposure to light are essential factors to consider when storing Ozempic.

Improper storage conditions, such as extreme heat or cold, can cause the medication to degrade, potentially reducing its effectiveness. Exposure to direct sunlight or excessive humidity may also damage the drug and compromise its chemical stability. It is essential to understand the specific storage requirements described on the product labeling and to consult healthcare professionals if uncertain.

CHAPTER 1

UNDERSTANDING OZEMPIC

Ozempic, also known as semaglutide, is a medicine used to treat type 2 diabetes. It belongs to a class of medicines called glucagon-like peptide-1 (GLP-1) receptor agonists. Ozempic is given as an injection once a week and works by mimicking the action of a hormone called GLP-1 in the body.

WHAT IS OZEMPIC?

Ozempic is a synthetic form of GLP-1, a hormone naturally produced in the intestines. GLP-1 has multiple functions in the body, but its main role is to stimulate the release of insulin from the pancreas after meals. Insulin is a hormone that helps regulate blood sugar levels by allowing glucose to enter cells, where it is used as energy or stored for future use.

In people with type 2 diabetes, there is a problem with insulin production, or the way the body uses insulin. This leads to high blood sugar levels, which can have adverse effects on various organs and systems of the body. Ozempic works by activating GLP-1 receptors in the pancreas, thereby promoting the release of insulin. This helps reduce blood sugar levels and improve blood sugar control.

HOW DOES OZEMPIC WORK?

Ozempic works through multiple mechanisms to regulate blood sugar and improve diabetes management. When injected, it binds to GLP-1 receptors in various tissues, including the pancreas, liver and brain.

The activation of these receptors triggers several physiological responses that contribute to its effectiveness.

1. Stimulation of insulin release: Ozempic enhances insulin release from pancreatic beta cells in response to high blood sugar levels. By increasing insulin secretion, it helps lower blood sugar levels after meals and reduces fasting blood sugar levels.

2. Inhibition of glucagon: glucagon is a hormone that has the opposite effect to insulin; this increases blood sugar levels. Ozempic suppresses the release of glucagon from pancreatic alpha cells, thereby reducing glucose production by the liver and preventing excessive release of glucose into the bloodstream.

3. Slowed Gastric Emptying: Ozempic slows stomach emptying, which helps regulate the rate at which glucose is absorbed into the bloodstream after a meal.

This helps reduce blood sugar spikes after meals and promotes more stable blood sugar control.

4. Increased satiety: GLP-1 agonists like Ozempic also act on the appetite centers of the brain, signaling a feeling of fullness and reducing appetite. This effect can lead to weight loss and help control calorie intake.

5. Preservation of pancreatic beta cells: Ozempic has shown its potential in preserving pancreatic beta cells, which are responsible for insulin production. By protecting these cells from damage or decline, Ozempic may help maintain long-term blood sugar control and delay the need for more intensive diabetes treatments.

BENEFITS AND RISKS OF OZEMPIC

Ozempic offers several benefits in the management of type 2 diabetes.

1. Improved Blood Glucose Control: By stimulating insulin secretion, inhibiting glucagon release and slowing gastric emptying, Ozempic helps regulate blood sugar levels, thereby reducing fasting and post-meal blood sugar levels. This helps improve blood sugar control and reduces the risk of diabetes-related complications.

2. Weight loss: One of the notable benefits of Ozempic is its potential to promote weight loss. GLP-1 receptor agonists have been shown to reduce appetite and food intake, leading to gradual and sustained weight loss. This can be beneficial for people with type 2 diabetes who often have difficulty managing their weight.

3. Cardiovascular benefits: Several studies have shown that Ozempic can reduce the risk of cardiovascular events in people with type 2 diabetes. These events include heart attacks, strokes, and cardiovascular death. The mechanisms behind these cardiovascular benefits are not fully understood, but they may involve favorable

effects on blood pressure, cholesterol levels, and arterial health.

4. Once a Week Dosage: Unlike some other diabetes medications that require daily administration, Ozempic is administered once a week. This convenience may improve adherence to the medication regimen and reduce the burden of daily self-injections.

Although Ozempic offers many benefits, it is essential to consider the potential risks and side effects associated with its use. Common side effects of Ozempic include nausea, vomiting, diarrhea, and constipation. These symptoms are usually mild and transient and often improve over time as the body adapts to the medication.

Rare but serious side effects may include pancreatitis, gallbladder disease, and thyroid tumors. It is important to discuss these potential risks with a healthcare professional before starting treatment with Ozempic. Additionally, patients should promptly report any unusual symptoms or concerns during treatment.

Ozempic is generally well tolerated, although individual responses may vary. The benefits and risks of using Ozempic should be carefully evaluated by healthcare providers on an individual basis, taking into account the patient's general health, lifestyle and other factors that may impact the effectiveness of treatment.

Overall, Ozempic is an effective and convenient treatment option for people with type 2 diabetes. It offers multiple benefits, including improved glycemic control, weight loss, and potential cardiovascular protection. As with any medication, it is important to be aware of both the benefits and potential risks associated with Ozempic and to consult healthcare professionals for advice and monitoring throughout the treatment journey.

CHAPTER 2

PRECAUTIONS AND CONTRAINDICATIONS

Ozempic is generally considered safe and effective for the management of type 2 diabetes. However, certain precautions and contraindications should be considered before using this medication. It is essential to discuss this with your healthcare professional to ensure Ozempic is the right treatment option for you.

WHO SHOULD NOT USE OZEMPIC?

Although Ozempic is suitable for many people with type 2 diabetes, some specific groups of people should avoid using this medication due to potential risks or contraindications. These include:

1. Type 1 diabetes: Ozempic is specifically indicated for the treatment of type 2 diabetes. It should not be used in people with type 1 diabetes, as it is not effective in regulating blood sugar in this population .

2. Allergy or hypersensitivity: If you have a known allergy or hypersensitivity to semaglutide or any of the ingredients in Ozempic, you should not use this medicine. Symptoms of an allergic reaction may include a rash, itching, swelling, dizziness, or difficulty breathing. If you experience any of these symptoms, seek medical attention immediately.

3. Diabetic ketoacidosis: Ozempic is not suitable for people with a history of diabetic ketoacidosis (DKA). DKA is a serious disease characterized by elevated levels of ketones in the blood, leading to metabolic imbalances and potential organ damage. If you have a history of DKA or are currently experiencing symptoms such as excessive thirst, frequent urination, abdominal pain, nausea, or vomiting, tell your doctor.

4. Pregnancy and breast-feeding: The safety of Ozempic during pregnancy and breast-feeding has not been established. It is recommended to avoid using this medication during pregnancy or if you plan to become pregnant. If you are breastfeeding, discuss the risks and benefits with your healthcare professional before starting Ozempic.

5. Renal Impairment: Ozempic has not been studied extensively in people with renal impairment. If you have moderate to severe kidney disease, your doctor may need to adjust the dosage or consider other treatment options.

6. Pancreatic disease: People with a history of pancreatitis should use caution when considering Ozempic. This medication may increase the risk of recurrent pancreatitis. If you have a history of pancreatitis or are currently experiencing abdominal pain, nausea, or vomiting, tell your healthcare professional.

7. Thyroid cancer: Some studies in rodents have suggested an increased risk of thyroid cancer with GLP-1 receptor agonists, including Ozempic. It is important to discuss any personal or family history of thyroid cancer with your healthcare professional before starting this medication.

8. Young Children: Ozempic is not recommended for use in children younger than 18 years, as its safety and effectiveness in this population have not been established.

It is essential to communicate your medical history and any existing conditions or concerns to your doctor to ensure that Ozempic is safe and appropriate for you.

IMPORTANT SAFETY INFORMATION

When using Ozempic, it is important to follow the prescribed dosage and administration instructions provided by your healthcare professional. Here are some important security considerations to keep in mind:

1. Injection technique: Ozempic is administered subcutaneously (under the skin) once a week. It is important to follow proper injection technique to ensure accurate dosing and minimize the risk of injection site reactions. Your healthcare professional will provide you with instructions on the correct administration technique.

2. Hypoglycemia: Although rare, hypoglycemia (low blood sugar) may occur when using Ozempic in combination with other diabetes medications that can cause hypoglycemia, such as insulin or sulfonylureas. Monitor your blood sugar regularly, especially when starting or adjusting treatment. Symptoms of

hypoglycemia may include sweating, shaking, fast heartbeat, dizziness, or confusion. If you experience these symptoms, treat hypoglycemia promptly by consuming a fast-acting source of glucose, such as glucose tablets or gel, fruit juice, or candy.

3. Pancreatitis: In rare cases, GLP-1 receptor agonists like Ozempic have been associated with pancreatitis, a potentially serious inflammation of the pancreas. If you experience severe and persistent abdominal pain, with or without vomiting, contact your healthcare professional immediately.

4. Gallbladder disease: GLP-1 receptor agonists may increase the risk of developing gallbladder disease or gallstones. If you experience symptoms such as abdominal pain, vomiting, or jaundice, tell your healthcare professional.

5. Hypersensitivity reactions: Some people may experience allergic reactions or hypersensitivity to

Ozempic. Seek medical attention if you develop signs of an allergic reaction, such as rash, itching, swelling, or difficulty breathing.

6. Cardiovascular Safety: Although Ozempic has demonstrated cardiovascular benefits in clinical trials, it is important to note that individual responses may vary. Monitor your cardiovascular health regularly and discuss any concerns with your healthcare professional.

7. Kidney failure: If you have kidney failure, your healthcare professional may need to adjust the dosage of Ozempic or consider other treatment options. It is essential to communicate any pre-existing kidney conditions or concerns to your doctor.

These are not exhaustive safety considerations, and it is important to consult your healthcare professional and carefully read the medication guide provided with Ozempic to ensure safe and effective use.

POTENTIAL DRUG INTERACTIONS

Ozempic may interact with other medicines, potentially affecting their effectiveness or increasing the risk of side effects. It is important to tell your doctor about all medications, including prescription, nonprescription, herbal, and supplements, that you take. Some medications that may interact with Ozempic include:

1. Insulin and insulin secretagogues: Combining Ozempic with insulin or drugs that stimulate insulin secretion (such as sulfonylureas) may increase the risk of hypoglycemia. Your doctor may need to adjust the dosage of these medications to minimize the risk of hypoglycemia.

2. Other GLP-1 receptor agonists: Concomitant use of multiple GLP-1 receptor agonists is not recommended, as this may increase the risk of adverse effects without additional benefits.

3. Warfarin and anticoagulants: Cases of increased international normalized ratio (INR) and bleeding events have been reported in people using GLP-1 receptor agonists with warfarin or other anticoagulant medications. Regular monitoring of INR and close monitoring for signs of bleeding is recommended if using these medications concurrently.

4. Oral medications: Some oral medications, such as antibiotics, may affect the absorption of Ozempic. Inform your doctor if you are prescribed other medications to ensure proper timing and minimize any potential interactions.

It is important to discuss any potential drug interactions with your healthcare professional or pharmacist. They can provide you with advice on the safe and effective use of Ozempic and any necessary adjustments to your medication regimen.

CHAPTER 3

First steps with Ozempic

Getting started with Ozempic involves understanding various aspects, including prescribing and dosing instructions, injection techniques, and dealing with common side effects. Ozempic is a medicine used to treat type 2 diabetes and its proper use is crucial for effective diabetes management.

PRESCRIPTION AND DOSAGE INSTRUCTIONS

Ozempic, also known by its generic name semaglutide, is a glucagon-like peptide-1 (GLP-1) receptor agonist. It is prescribed to people with type 2 diabetes to help regulate blood sugar levels. Before starting Ozempic, it is essential to have a thorough discussion with your healthcare professional. They will consider factors such as your general health, medical history, and current medications to determine if Ozempic is the right choice for you.

Ozempic dosage is usually administered once a week. Your healthcare professional will prescribe the appropriate dose, which is usually started at a lower level and adjusted if necessary. The medication comes in a pre-filled pen, making it easier to self-administer at home.

INJECTION TECHNIQUES AND BEST PRACTICES

Ozempic is administered subcutaneously, which means it is injected under the skin. Proper injection technique is essential to ensure that the medication is administered effectively. Here are some key steps for injecting Ozempic:

1. Preparation: Wash your hands thoroughly before handling the Ozempic pen. Check the medicine for any discoloration or particles. If you notice anything unusual, do not use it and consult your healthcare professional.

2. Injection site: Choose a clean, dry area on your abdomen for the injection. Rotate injection sites to prevent lipoatrophy or lipohypertrophy – conditions that affect drug absorption.

3. Administration: Follow the instructions provided by your healthcare professional to use the pre-filled pen. The injection process is relatively simple and involves a quick subcutaneous injection.

4. Disposal: Safely dispose of the used Ozempic pen in accordance with local regulations. Do not share your pen with others.

Remember to consult your healthcare professional if you have any concerns or questions regarding the injection process. They can provide you with personalized advice based on your individual needs.

COMMON SIDE EFFECTS AND THEIR MANAGEMENT

Like any medicine, Ozempic can cause side effects. Understanding these potential side effects and knowing how to manage them is crucial for a safe and effective treatment experience. Common side effects of Ozempic include:

1. Nausea: Some people may experience mild nausea, especially when they first start taking Ozempic. This side effect often improves over time. Taking medicine with food can help relieve nausea.

2. Injection site reactions: Redness, swelling, or itching at the injection site may occur. Rotating injection sites and using proper injection techniques can minimize these reactions.

3. Gastrointestinal problems: Diarrhea and constipation may occur. Staying hydrated and eating a balanced, fiber-rich diet can help manage these symptoms.

4. Hypoglycemia: Ozempic, when used in combination with other diabetes medications such as insulin or sulfonylureas, may increase the risk of hypoglycemia. Be

aware of the signs of hypoglycemia, such as shaking, sweating and confusion, and have a plan in place to manage it.

It is essential to report any serious or persistent side effects to your doctor promptly. They can adjust your treatment plan if necessary or provide additional advice to address specific concerns.

CHAPTER 4

CONSERVATION D'OZEMPIC

It is essential to store Ozempic appropriately to maintain its effectiveness and ensure its safety for use. Understanding appropriate temperature and environmental conditions, handling and transportation guidelines, as well as knowing shelf life and expiration dates, are essential aspects of responsible medication management.

APPROPRIATE TEMPERATURE AND ENVIRONMENTAL CONDITIONS

Ozempic, like many medications, is sensitive to temperature and environmental conditions. Improper storage can cause a loss of potency, making the medication less effective. Here are the main considerations for storing Ozempic:

1. Refrigeration: Ozempic pens should be stored in a refrigerator between 36°F and 46°F (2°C to 8°C). It is essential to maintain the medication within this temperature range to prevent degradation.

2. Avoid freezing: Freezing can damage the structure of the medicine. Make sure that the Ozempic pen does not come into direct contact with the freezer compartment. If the medicine freezes, it should be thrown away and a new pen used.

3. Protect from light: Ozempic pens should be stored in their original packaging to protect them from light. Exposure to light may affect the stability of the drug.

4. Do not store in the bathroom: Avoid storing Ozempic in the bathroom or other humid environments. Moisture may compromise the integrity of the medication. The refrigerator provides a controlled, dry environment for storage.

5. Keep out of reach of children: Keep Ozempic out of reach of children and pets. This medicine should be treated with the same caution as any other potentially harmful substance.

By adhering to these storage guidelines, you can ensure that your Ozempic remains potent and safe to use for the entire prescribed duration.

HANDLING AND TRANSPORT OZEMPIC

Proper handling and transportation of Ozempic is essential to avoid damage to the medication and maintain its effectiveness. Whether you're at home or on the go, it's essential to follow these guidelines:

1. Gentle handling: When handling Ozempic pens, be gentle to avoid unnecessary agitation. Rough handling may affect the stability of the drug.

2. Store in its original packaging: When transporting Ozempic, it is advisable to keep it in its original packaging. This provides an extra layer of protection and helps protect the medicine from light.

3. Use a cooler bag for traveling: If you must travel with Ozempic, especially in warmer climates, consider using a cooler bag with ice packs. Make sure the medicine does

not come into direct contact with the ice packs to avoid freezing.

4. Plan an extended trip: If you are planning an extended trip, discuss your travel plans with your healthcare professional in advance. They can provide you with advice on how to efficiently store and transport Ozempic during your trip.

5. Emergency Preparedness: Have a plan in case of an emergency, such as a power outage. If a power outage occurs and you are unable to access your refrigerated Ozempic, consult your healthcare professional for advice on using a new pen.

SHELF LIFE AND EXPIRY DATE

Understanding the shelf life and expiration date of Ozempic is essential for its safe and effective use. Here are the key points to consider:

1. Check the expiration date: Each Ozempic pen comes with an expiration date printed on the package. It is crucial to check this date before using the medicine. Using Ozempic after its expiration date may be ineffective and potentially dangerous.

2. Store unopened pens properly: Unopened Ozempic pens should be stored in the refrigerator until their expiration date. Always check the packaging for any signs of damage before use.

3. Use opened pens promptly: Once an Ozempic pen has been opened, it can be stored at room temperature (up

to 86°F or 30°C) for up to 56 days. Throw away any unused medicine after this time.

4. Do not freeze: Avoid freezing Ozempic pens, as this may compromise their effectiveness. If a pen has been frozen, it should be thrown away and a new pen used.

5. Dispose of expired medications properly: If you have expired Ozempic pens, dispose of them according to local drug disposal regulations. Do not throw them in the trash, as this may pose environmental risks.

Check the expiration dates of your medications regularly and consult your doctor if you have any concerns or questions regarding storage or use. They can provide you with personalized advice based on your specific situation.

CHAPTER 5

INTEGRATE OZEMPIC INTO YOUR ROUTINE

Incorporating Ozempic into your routine is an important step in effectively managing type 2 diabetes. This process involves developing a consistent injection schedule, finding practical ways to remember doses, and managing lifestyle and diet changes to optimize the benefits of Ozempic. Let's look at each aspect to provide comprehensive information on seamlessly integrating Ozempic into your daily life.

DEVELOP A CONSISTENT INJECTION SCHEDULE

Establishing a consistent injection schedule is paramount to the success of Ozempic in the management of diabetes. Consistency ensures that you receive the medication as prescribed, maintaining stable blood sugar levels. Here's a guide to help you develop a routine:

1. Align with daily activities: Choose a time for your Ozempic injection that fits your daily routine. Many people find it convenient to administer the medication in the morning or evening, depending on their personal preferences and lifestyle.

2. Set alarms or reminders: Use alarms or reminders on your phone to notify you when it's time for your Ozempic injection. This helps create a routine and reduces the risk of forgetting a dose.

3. Incorporate with meals or at bedtime:*l Some people prefer to take Ozempic with a specific meal or at bedtime. Discuss this option with your healthcare professional to make sure it fits into your treatment plan.

4. Consistency over flexibility: Although Ozempic has a flexible dosing window, look for consistency. Injecting the medication at the same time each day helps regulate its effectiveness and contributes to better blood sugar control.

5. Travel Considerations: If you travel frequently or have an irregular schedule, plan your injection times accordingly. Consult your healthcare professional for advice on adjusting your schedule while traveling.

By incorporating Ozempic into your routine at a consistent time, you create a habit that promotes adherence to your treatment plan, improving the overall effectiveness of the medication.

TIPS FOR MEMORIZING DOSES

Remembering to take your doses of Ozempic regularly is essential for optimal diabetes management. Here are some practical tips to help you remember your doses:

1. Use medication apps: Smartphone apps designed for medication management can be invaluable. Set up reminders through these apps to receive notifications when it's time for your Ozempic injection.

2. Pair it with another activity: Pair your Ozempic injection with another daily activity, such as brushing your teeth or eating a meal. This pairing creates a mental connection, which makes memorization easier.

3. Visual reminders: Place visual reminders in prominent places. This could be a post-it note on your refrigerator or a calendar marker marking your injection days. Visual cues can reinforce this habit.

4. Involve a support system: Let family members, friends, or coworkers know about your Ozempic schedule. They can provide encouragement and gentle reminders, creating a supportive environment.

5. Establish a routine: Make taking Ozempic part of your daily routine. The more seamlessly it fits into your

lifestyle, the less likely you are to forget doses. Consistency of routine provides a strong foundation for medication adherence.

6. Use pill boxes: Although Ozempic is administered using injector pens, using a pill box can help you follow your treatment schedule. Place the pens in the weekly organizer to visually track your injections.

MANAGING LIFESTYLE AND DIETARY CHANGES

Incorporating Ozempic into your routine also involves managing lifestyle and diet changes that may accompany your diabetes management plan. Ozempic works most effectively when combined with a healthy lifestyle. Consider the following aspects:

1. Dietary adjustments: Consult a registered dietitian or your healthcare professional to make appropriate dietary adjustments. Ozempic is most effective when supplemented with a balanced diet that supports stable blood sugar levels.

2. Regular physical activity: Integrate regular physical activity into your routine. Exercise may improve the effectiveness of Ozempic and help with overall diabetes management. Discuss appropriate exercise options with your healthcare professional.

3. Hydration: Make sure you stay adequately hydrated. Proper hydration supports the body's metabolic processes and can contribute to the overall effectiveness of diabetes management.

4. Alcohol Consumption: If you consume alcohol, do so in moderation and be aware of its impact on blood sugar levels. Discuss alcohol use with your healthcare professional to make sure it fits into your treatment plan.

5. Regular monitoring: Monitor your blood sugar regularly as advised by your healthcare professional. This helps monitor the impact of Ozempic and allows you to adjust your treatment plan if necessary.

6. Stress Management: Explore stress management techniques, as stress can impact blood sugar levels. Practices such as meditation, deep breathing exercises, or taking up hobbies can contribute to a balanced lifestyle.

7. Regular Follow-ups: Schedule regular follow-up appointments with your healthcare professional to evaluate the effectiveness of Ozempic and make any necessary adjustments to your treatment plan. Communication with your healthcare team is crucial to successful diabetes management.

By proactively managing lifestyle and diet changes, you create an environment that supports the effectiveness of Ozempic. These adjustments work in tandem with the medication to help you achieve and maintain stable blood sugar levels.

CHAPTER 6

MONITOR YOUR PROGRESS

Monitoring your progress is an essential aspect of effectively managing type 2 diabetes, especially when you incorporate medications like Ozempic into your treatment plan. This process involves regular monitoring of blood sugar levels, adjusting doses if necessary, and promptly reporting any side effects or concerns to your healthcare professional. In this comprehensive guide, we'll explore each of these components to provide an in-depth understanding of how to track your progress while using Ozempic.

REGULAR MONITORING OF BLOOD GLUCOSE

1. Importance of Blood Glucose Monitoring:

Regular blood sugar monitoring is the cornerstone of diabetes management. It provides valuable information about how your blood sugar is controlled and allows you to make informed decisions about your treatment plan. Monitoring is especially crucial when using medications like Ozempic, which aim to regulate blood sugar levels over time.

2. Monitoring frequency:

The frequency of blood sugar monitoring may vary depending on individual circumstances and stage of diabetes management. In the early stages of using Ozempic, your healthcare professional may recommend more frequent monitoring to assess its impact. Over time, as stability is achieved, monitoring may become less frequent, but it should remain an integral part of your routine.

3. Blood Glucose Monitoring Methods:

There are different methods of monitoring blood sugar, including:

Blood Glucose Meters: These portable devices allow you to check your blood sugar at home. Follow the instructions that came with your meter to get accurate results.

Continuous Glucose Monitoring (CGM): CGM systems provide real-time data on your blood sugar levels throughout the day. They involve a small sensor placed under the skin that measures glucose levels in the interstitial fluid.

Hemoglobin A1c test: This blood test provides an average of your blood sugar level over the past two to three months. This is usually done every three to six months.

4. Interpretation of results:

Understand the blood sugar target ranges set by your doctor. Interpretation of results may involve considering factors such as fasting blood sugar, postprandial (after meal) blood sugar, and general trends. Consistently high or low readings may indicate the need to adjust your treatment plan.

ADJUST DOSAGES AS NEEDED

1. Collaborative approach with healthcare provider:

Dosage adjustments of Ozempic should always be done in conjunction with your healthcare professional. They will take into account various factors, including your blood sugar levels, your general health and any side effects you may be experiencing. Do not make dosage adjustments independently; Always seek professional advice.

2. Initial dosage and titration:

Ozempic is often started at a lower dose to allow your body to adapt. The dosage may be increased gradually depending on your response to the medication. The titration schedule is determined by your healthcare professional to achieve the desired glycemic control.

3. Blood Glucose Trends:

Regular monitoring of blood glucose plays a crucial role in determining whether dosage adjustments are necessary. If you regularly experience high or low blood sugar levels, this information is essential so that your doctor can make informed decisions about changing your Ozempic dosage.

4. Report lifestyle changes:

Lifestyle changes, such as changes in diet, exercise habits, or stress levels, can impact your blood sugar control. Communicate any significant changes in your lifestyle to your healthcare professional so that they can assess whether adjustments to your Ozempic dosage are necessary.

5. Side effects and dosage adjustments:

If you experience any side effects, particularly persistent or serious, tell your healthcare professional promptly. Some side effects may indicate that the dosage needs to be adjusted. Managing side effects is essential to ensure your treatment plan is both effective and well-tolerated.

6. Regular follow-up appointments:

Schedule regular follow-up appointments with your healthcare professional to discuss your progress. These appointments allow for a complete review of your blood sugar levels, potential adjustments to your Ozempic dose, and the opportunity to answer any questions or concerns you may have.

REPORTING SIDE EFFECTS OR CONCERNS

1. Recognize side effects:

It is essential to be aware of the potential side effects associated with Ozempic. Common side effects may include nausea, injection site reactions, or gastrointestinal problems. However, everyone's reaction to medications is unique, and some people may experience rare or unexpected side effects.

2. When to report side effects:

Report side effects promptly to your healthcare professional. If you experience serious or persistent side effects, do not wait for your next appointment. An immediate report allows your doctor to assess the situation, determine if adjustments are needed, or explore alternative treatment options.

3. Communication with the care team:

Open communication with your healthcare team is essential for effective diabetes management. Discuss any concerns or questions you have about Ozempic during your appointments. Your healthcare professional is there to support you and ensure your treatment plan aligns with your overall health goals.

4. Emergency Situations:

In rare cases, some side effects may require urgent attention. If you experience symptoms such as difficulty breathing, severe allergic reactions, or other signs of a medical emergency, seek medical attention immediately.

5. Document side effects:

Keep track of any side effects you experience, along with the date and time they occurred. This documentation can help your doctor evaluate trends and make informed decisions about your treatment plan.

6. Adjustments to treatment plan:

Depending on the nature and severity of side effects, your healthcare professional may recommend adjustments to your treatment plan. This could involve changing Ozempic dosage, exploring alternative medications, or implementing additional strategies to manage specific side effects.

CHAPTER 7

OVERCOME CHALLENGES AND TRAPS

Overcoming challenges and pitfalls is an integral part of managing type 2 diabetes, and this is especially true when you incorporate medications like Ozempic into your treatment plan. This guide looks at strategies for managing injection anxiety, solving common injection problems, and managing unwanted weight changes. Understanding and addressing these challenges can contribute to a more successful and comfortable experience with Ozempic.

DEALING WITH ANXIETY BY INJECTION

1. Understanding injection anxiety:

Injection anxiety is a common concern among people using medications that require self-administration, like Ozempic. Recognizing and understanding this anxiety is essential to responding to it effectively.

2. Educate yourself:

Knowledge is a powerful tool for managing anxiety. Learn about the purpose of Ozempic, how it works in your body, and the benefits it offers. Understanding the positive impact on managing your diabetes can help ease anxiety.

3. Start slowly:

If you feel anxious about injections, consider starting slowly. Start with smaller steps, like practicing with an empty pen or watching video tutorials on proper injection techniques. Gradually build your confidence as you become more familiar with the process.

4. Use support systems:

Seek support from friends, family, or support groups. Share your concerns and feelings about injection anxiety. Sometimes talking about it with others who have had similar experiences can provide valuable information and emotional support.

5. Mind-Body Techniques:

Explore mindfulness and relaxation techniques to manage anxiety. Techniques such as deep breathing, meditation, or guided imagery can help calm your mind and reduce anxiety associated with injections.

6. Professional assistance:

If anxiety persists, consider seeking professional help. A mental health professional, such as a counselor or psychologist, can work with you to develop coping strategies specifically tailored to your needs.

7. Desensitization Techniques:

Gradual exposure to the injection process, called desensitization, can be helpful. This involves gradually increasing your comfort level with the steps involved in administering Ozempic until the process becomes more routine.

8. Reward System:

Set up a reward system for yourself after each successful injection. This could be a small treat, a moment of relaxation or any positive reinforcement to associate the injection process with positive experiences.

9. Open communication with healthcare provider:

Share your anxiety with your healthcare professional. They can offer advice, resources and reassurance. In some cases, they may adjust your treatment plan or explore other medications if injection anxiety becomes a significant barrier.

TROUBLESHOOTING COMMON INJECTION PROBLEMS

1. Injection site reactions:

Common reactions at the injection site may include redness, swelling, or itching. To minimize these reactions, ensure proper injection technique, alternate injection sites, and use alcohol swabs to clean the injection site before administration.

2. Bruising:

Bruising may occur if the needle touches a blood vessel. To reduce the risk, avoid injecting directly into visible veins and use the correct needle length. If bruising persists, consult your healthcare professional for advice on adjusting your injection technique.

3. Leak or drip:

Sometimes a small amount of medicine may leak out after the injection. To avoid this, hold the pen in place for a few seconds after injection to allow the medicine to be absorbed. If the leak persists, contact your healthcare professional for further advice.

4. Clogged needle:

If you have difficulty using the needle or notice that it is clogged, do not use force. Replace the needle and make sure it is securely attached before giving the injection. If problems persist, contact your doctor or pharmacist for help.

5. Pen malfunction:

In rare cases, the Ozempic pen may malfunction. If you notice any problems with the pen, such as difficulty turning the dose selector or problems with the injection mechanism, contact your healthcare professional or pharmaceutical company for advice.

6. Pain during injection:

If you feel pain during the injection, make sure the needle is inserted at the correct angle and that you are using a new, sharp needle. If pain persists, see your doctor to explore potential causes and solutions.

7. Allergic reactions:

Although rare, allergic reactions to Ozempic can occur. If you experience symptoms such as rash, itching, swelling, or difficulty breathing, seek medical attention immediately. Report any allergic reactions to your healthcare professional promptly.

8. Injection site infections:

Maintain good hygiene when administering Ozempic to prevent infections. If you notice signs of infection, such as redness, warmth, or pus at the injection site, contact your healthcare professional for advice.

RESPONDING TO UNWANTED WEIGHT CHANGES

1. Understand weight changes with Ozempic:

Weight changes, both gains and losses, may occur with the use of Ozempic. It is essential to understand that individual responses vary and weight changes can be influenced by a variety of factors.

2. Diet and Exercise:

Evaluate your diet and exercise habits. Weight changes could be linked to lifestyle factors. Consult a registered dietitian to ensure your diet supports your overall health and diabetes management goals.

3. See a healthcare provider:

If you notice significant, unexplained weight changes, consult your healthcare professional. They can assess whether the changes are related to Ozempic, other medicines, or underlying health problems.

4. Nutritional Tips:

Work with a healthcare professional, such as a dietitian, to receive personalized nutritional advice. They can help you make informed choices that align with your diabetes management goals and support a healthy weight.

5. Hormonal factors:

Understand that hormonal factors can influence weight changes. Ozempic works by affecting the appetite control center in the brain, which may impact food intake. If you have concerns about weight changes, discuss them with your healthcare professional.

6. Regular monitoring:

Monitor your weight regularly and report any significant changes to your healthcare professional. Keeping a diary of your weight can provide valuable information for assessing trends and making informed decisions about your treatment plan.

7. Changes in body composition:

Consider that weight changes don't just reflect changes in fat. Ozempic may cause changes in body composition, including a reduction in fat mass and an increase in lean mass. This can help improve metabolic health.

8. Lifestyle Changes:

If you're concerned about weight changes, work with your doctor to explore lifestyle changes. This may include adjustments to diet, exercise programs, or other factors that may contribute to a healthy weight.

9. Psychosocial factors:

Recognize the potential impact of psychosocial factors on weight changes. Stress, emotional well-being and mental health can influence eating habits and weight. Seek support from mental health professionals if needed.

BONUS CHAPTER

FAQ

1. What is Ozempic used for?

   Ozempic is used to treat type 2 diabetes in adults and helps improve blood sugar control.

2. How is Ozempic administered?

   Ozempic is given by subcutaneous injection, usually once a week.

3. Can I self-administer Ozempic at home?

   Yes, Ozempic comes in a pre-filled pen form, allowing for convenient self-administration at home.

4. What is the recommended dosage for Ozempic?

The recommended dosage of Ozempic is determined by your healthcare professional and is often started at a lower level, adjusted gradually as needed.

5. Are there any common side effects related to Ozempic?

Common side effects may include nausea, injection site reactions, and gastrointestinal problems. Consult your healthcare professional for more information.

6. How does Ozempic work in the body?

Ozempic is a GLP-1 receptor agonist that helps regulate blood sugar levels by increasing insulin production and reducing glucagon secretion.

7. Can Ozempic be used with other diabetes medications?

Yes, Ozempic is often used in combination with other diabetes medications to achieve better blood sugar control.

8. What should I do if I miss a dose of Ozempic?

If you miss a dose, give it as soon as you remember. Consult your healthcare professional for advice on missed doses.

9. How long does it take for Ozempic to start working?

Ozempic may start to work within a few days, but individual responses may vary. Consult your healthcare professional for personalized information.

10. Can I travel with Ozempic?

Yes, you can travel with Ozempic. Ensure proper storage and consult your healthcare professional for any travel-related considerations.

11. Is refrigeration necessary to store Ozempic?

Yes, Ozempic should be stored in the refrigerator between 36°F and 46°F (2°C to 8°C).

12. Can Ozempic cause hypoglycemia?

Although Ozempic itself does not cause hypoglycemia, using it in combination with other diabetes medications may increase the risk. Be aware of the symptoms and consult your healthcare professional.

13. How often should I monitor my blood sugar levels while using Ozempic?

The frequency of blood glucose monitoring may vary. Follow your healthcare professional's recommendations for monitoring while using Ozempic.

14. Can I adjust the dose of Ozempic myself?

No, dosage adjustments should be made in consultation with your healthcare professional. Do not make independent changes to your dosage.

15. Is Ozempic safe to use during pregnancy?

Consult your healthcare professional if you are pregnant, planning to become pregnant, or breastfeeding before using Ozempic.

16. Can I drink alcohol while using Ozempic?

Moderate alcohol consumption may be acceptable, but discuss it with your doctor to make sure it fits into your treatment plan.

17. Are there any dietary restrictions when using Ozempic?

Although there are no specific dietary restrictions, consult a registered dietitian to ensure your diet supports your overall health and diabetes management goals.

18. Can I use Ozempic if I have kidney problems?

Consult your healthcare professional for personalized advice if you have kidney problems before using Ozempic.

19. What should I do if I have injection site reactions?

If you experience injection site reactions, follow proper injection techniques, alternate sites, and consult your healthcare professional if problems persist.

20. What is the shelf life of an unopened Ozempic pen?

The shelf life of an unopened Ozempic pen is specified on the packaging. Always check the expiration date before use.

21. Can I share my Ozempic pen with other people?

No, Ozempic pens should not be shared. Each pen is intended for individual use only.

22. What is the most common misconception about Ozempic?

A common misconception is that Ozempic causes weight gain. In reality, it can lead to weight loss or changes in body composition.

23. Can Ozempic be used in children with diabetes?

Ozempic is not usually prescribed to children. Consult your healthcare professional for appropriate treatments for pediatric diabetes.

24. Does Ozempic require a prescription?

Yes, Ozempic is a prescription medication. Consult your healthcare professional to determine if this is appropriate for your diabetes management.

25. Can I inject Ozempic into any part of my body?

Ozempic is usually injected into the abdomen. Consult your healthcare professional for appropriate injection site recommendations.

26. How can I manage nausea, a common side effect of Ozempic?

Taking Ozempic with food can help manage nausea. Consult your healthcare professional for personalized advice.

27. Does Ozempic interact with other medications?

Tell your healthcare professional about all medications you are taking to assess potential interactions with Ozempic.

28. What should I do if I have an allergic reaction to Ozempic?

Seek immediate medical attention if you have symptoms of an allergic reaction, such as rash, swelling, or difficulty breathing.

29. Can I exercise while using Ozempic?

Yes, regular exercise is encouraged. Consult your healthcare professional for personalized exercise recommendations.

30. What is the role of Ozempic in a comprehensive diabetes management plan?

Ozempic is a GLP-1 receptor agonist that helps regulate blood sugar levels and is often used as part of a comprehensive diabetes management plan.

31. How long does each Ozempic injection last?

The injection process is relatively quick and usually takes a few seconds. Follow the instructions provided by your healthcare professional.

32. Is it normal to experience changes in appetite with Ozempic?

Appetite changes are a possible side effect. Consult your healthcare professional if you have concerns about changes in appetite.

33. Can I use Ozempic if I have a history of pancreatitis?

Discuss your medical history, including pancreatitis, with your healthcare professional before using Ozempic.

34. Is it safe to use Ozempic if I have a history of heart disease?

Consult your healthcare professional to evaluate the safety of using Ozempic based on your individual medical history.

35. What is the main mechanism of action of Ozempic?

Ozempic acts as a GLP-1 receptor agonist, enhancing insulin production and reducing glucagon secretion.

36. Can I take Ozempic if I have liver problems?

Discuss your liver health with your healthcare professional before using Ozempic.

37. Is it common to experience dizziness as a side effect of Ozempic?

Dizziness is not a common side effect, but if you experience it, consult your healthcare professional.

38. Can Ozempic be used as a stand-alone treatment for diabetes?

Ozempic is often used in combination with other diabetes medications for comprehensive care.

39. Is Ozempic effective in reducing HbA1c levels?

Yes, Ozempic has been shown to be effective in reducing HbA1c levels in clinical studies.

40. How long after starting Ozempic can I expect to see an improvement in my blood sugar levels?

Individual responses vary, but some people may see improvements within a few days. Consult your healthcare professional for personalized information.

41. Can I use Ozempic if I have a busy lifestyle and irregular meal times?

Ozempic has a flexible dosing window, making it suitable for people with busy lifestyles. Consult your healthcare professional for advice.

42. What should I do if I accidentally inject more than the prescribed dose of Ozempic?

Contact your healthcare professional or seek medical attention if you accidentally inject more than the prescribed dose.

43. Is it common to experience fatigue with Ozempic?

Fatigue is a less common side effect, but if you experience it, consult your healthcare professional.

44. Can Ozempic be used in older people with diabetes?

Ozempic can be used in older people, but individual health status should be taken into account. Consult your healthcare professional for personalized advice.

45. Can I take over-the-counter medications while using Ozempic?

Tell your healthcare professional about all medications, including over-the-counter medications, to evaluate potential interactions with Ozempic.

46. Can Ozempic be used in people with a history of eating disorders?

Consult your healthcare professional to discuss the use of Ozempic in people with a history of eating disorders.

47. How long does the effect of each dose of Ozempic last in the body?

The duration of effect may vary, but Ozempic is designed for once-weekly administration. Consult your healthcare professional for personalized information.

48. Can I drink herbal teas while using Ozempic?

Herbal teas are generally okay, but consult your doctor for advice on specific food choices.

49. Is Ozempic suitable for people with a history of depression?

Discuss your mental health history with your healthcare professional before using Ozempic.

50. What should I do if I experience persistent stomach pain while using Ozempic?

If you experience persistent stomach pain, see your doctor for thorough evaluation and advice.

CHAPTER 8

OZEMPIC AND DIABETES MANAGEMENT

Ozempic, a GLP-1 receptor agonist, has proven to be a valuable tool in the overall management of type 2 diabetes. In this in-depth exploration, we will examine how Ozempic fits into diabetes treatment plans, compare its effectiveness to other diabetes medications and explore the benefits of combining Ozempic with other treatment methods. Understanding Ozempic's role in diabetes management is crucial for people looking for effective, personalized strategies to control their blood sugar levels.

HOW OZEMPIC FITS INTO DIABETES TREATMENT PLANS

1. Mechanism of action:

Ozempic, or semaglutide, is a glucagon-like peptide-1 (GLP-1) receptor agonist. It mimics the action of GLP-1, a natural hormone that stimulates insulin release, reduces glucagon secretion and slows gastric emptying. This multidimensional approach contributes to better blood sugar control.

2. Blood sugar regulation:

Ozempic primarily targets postprandial (after meals) blood sugar levels, making it effective in reducing the spikes that often occur after eating. By improving insulin secretion and suppressing glucagon release, it helps maintain more stable blood sugar levels throughout the day.

3. Dosage once a week:

A notable feature of Ozempic is its once-a-week dosing regimen. This convenience improves adherence to the treatment plan, providing individuals with a manageable and consistent approach to diabetes management.

4. Benefits of Weight Management:

Ozempic has demonstrated weight loss benefits in addition to its impact on blood sugar control. This may be particularly beneficial for people with type 2 diabetes who may also be overweight or obese.

5. Flexible dosing window:

Ozempic offers a flexible dosing window, allowing individuals to administer the medication at a time that fits their lifestyle. This flexibility improves the practicality of integrating Ozempic into daily routines.

6. Cardiovascular Benefits:

Clinical studies have indicated cardiovascular benefits associated with the use of Ozempic. These benefits include a reduced risk of major adverse cardiovascular events in people with type 2 diabetes and established cardiovascular disease.

7. Complementary to lifestyle changes:

Ozempic is often prescribed as part of a comprehensive approach to diabetes management, which includes lifestyle modifications such as dietary changes, regular exercise, and weight management.

8. Individualized Treatment Plans:

The incorporation of Ozempic into diabetes treatment plans is highly individualized. Healthcare providers evaluate factors such as overall health, treatment goals and individual response to determine the most effective and personalized approach.

COMPARISON OF OZEMPIC TO OTHER DIABETES DRUGS

1. GLP-1 receptor agonists compared to other drugs:

Ozempic belongs to the class of GLP-1 receptor agonists, which includes drugs like liraglutide and dulaglutide. These drugs share a similar mechanism of action, promoting the release of insulin and reducing blood sugar levels. Compared to other diabetes medications such as sulfonylureas or metformin, GLP-1 receptor agonists offer different benefits and considerations.

2. Weight Loss Benefits:

A distinguishing factor of GLP-1 receptor agonists, including Ozempic, is their association with weight loss. This contrasts with some other diabetes medications that may be weight neutral or associated with weight gain.

3. Insulin Sensitivity:

GLP-1 receptor agonists improve insulin sensitivity, making them effective in people with insulin resistance, a common feature of type 2 diabetes. This contrasts with medications like metformin, which mainly target insulin resistance through different mechanisms.

4. Side effect profiles:

Each class of diabetes medications has its own side effect profile. For example, sulfonylureas may be associated with hypoglycemia, while GLP-1 receptor agonists may have side effects such as nausea. The choice of medication is often influenced by individual health considerations and tolerability.

5. Cardiovascular Considerations:

GLP-1 receptor agonists, including Ozempic, have demonstrated cardiovascular benefits in clinical studies. This cardiovascular protection sets them apart from some other diabetes medications.

6. Combination Therapies:

The choice of diabetes medications is often influenced by the need for combination therapies. Ozempic can be used in combination with other drug classes, providing healthcare providers flexibility in tailoring treatment plans.

7. Individual response:

Individual responses to diabetes medications vary. Some people may respond more favorably to GLP-1 receptor agonists like Ozempic, while others may have better results with different classes of medications. The choice often involves a collaborative decision-making process between the individual and their health care provider.

COMBINATION OZEMPIC WITH OTHER TREATMENT METHODS

1. Lifestyle Changes:

The synergy between Ozempic and lifestyle modifications is the cornerstone of effective diabetes management. Combining the medication with dietary changes, regular exercise, and weight management efforts improves overall blood sugar control and contributes to better long-term results.

2. Dietary Approaches:

Ozempic complements dietary approaches focused on balanced nutrition, portion control and carbohydrate management. Working with a registered dietitian can help individuals create meal plans that align with both their diabetes management goals and what Ozempic does.

3. Regular exercise:

Physical activity is an integral part of diabetes management. Regular exercise not only helps manage weight but also improves insulin sensitivity. Combining Ozempic with a consistent exercise routine contributes to a holistic approach to diabetes care.

4. Continuous Blood Glucose Monitoring:

Integrating continuous glucose monitoring (CGM) into diabetes management can provide real-time blood glucose data. This information is valuable for adjusting Ozempic dosages and making informed decisions regarding lifestyle modifications.

5. Personalized Treatment Plans:

The effectiveness of combining Ozempic with other treatment methods lies in creating personalized treatment plans. Healthcare providers assess individual needs, preferences and responses to design a comprehensive, sustainable approach to diabetes management.

6. Drug Combinations:

Ozempic may be used in combination with other diabetes medications, such as metformin or insulin, to achieve optimal blood sugar control. The choice of combination therapy depends on individual factors and the overall therapeutic strategy.

7. Regular monitoring and adjustments:

Continuous blood sugar monitoring, combined with regular follow-up appointments with healthcare providers, allows for timely adjustments to treatment plans. This proactive approach ensures that the combination of Ozempic and other treatment methods remains effective over time.

8. Education and Support:

Providing individuals with diabetes education and ongoing support is essential when combining Ozempic with other treatment methods. Providing individuals with knowledge about their health conditions, medications, and lifestyle strategies promotes active participation in their own care.

CHAPTER 9

Ozempic and weight loss

Ozempic, a GLP-1 receptor agonist originally designed to manage type 2 diabetes, has gained attention for its weight loss benefits. In this comprehensive exploration, we'll examine how Ozempic affects weight, compare its effectiveness to other weight loss methods, and address concerns related to weight loss while taking Ozempic. Understanding the mechanisms and implications of weight loss with Ozempic is essential for people seeking both diabetes management and potential improvement in their overall weight.

HOW OZEMPIC AFFECTS WEIGHT

1. Weight Loss Mechanism:

The weight loss effects of Ozempic are attributed to its impact on several physiological processes. As a GLP-1 receptor agonist, Ozempic increases the feeling of fullness (fullness), reduces appetite, and slows gastric emptying. These actions collectively contribute to a decrease in calorie intake and, therefore, weight loss.

2. Appetite regulation:

Ozempic influences the appetite control center in the brain, leading to a reduction in feelings of hunger. This effect may be particularly beneficial for people who struggle with overeating or have difficulty adhering to dietary restrictions.

3. Gastrointestinal effects:

The medication also slows the rate at which the stomach empties its contents into the small intestine.

This delayed gastric emptying extends the period during which nutrients are absorbed, contributing to a prolonged feeling of fullness and a reduction in overall food consumption.

4. Impact on body composition:

Beyond weight loss, Ozempic has demonstrated favorable effects on body composition. Studies suggest a reduction in fat mass and an increase in lean mass, highlighting the potential metabolic improvements associated with its use.

5. Reduction in calorie intake:

By addressing both sides of the energy balance equation – reducing appetite and slowing nutrient absorption – Ozempic creates a calorie deficit, which is fundamental to weight loss. The gradual and lasting nature of this weight loss distinguishes it from faster, but often less sustainable, approaches.

6. Individual Variability:

It is important to note that individual responses to Ozempic may vary. Although weight loss is a common outcome, the degree of weight loss may differ among individuals. Factors such as baseline weight, lifestyle and genetic predispositions can influence individual responses.

7. Additional effects on diabetes:

Weight loss associated with Ozempic is often considered a positive side effect, especially for people with type 2 diabetes, who may also benefit from improved insulin sensitivity and blood sugar control.

COMPARISON OF OZEMPIC TO OTHER WEIGHT LOSS METHODS

1. Comparison with diet and exercise:

Ozempic's approach to weight loss differs from traditional methods like diet and exercise. While lifestyle modifications remain crucial parts of a healthy weight management plan, Ozempic can provide additional support, particularly for people struggling with lasting changes in their eating habits and physical activity.

2. Unique mechanism of action:

Ozempic's unique mechanism of action sets it apart from many weight loss medications and interventions. Rather than relying solely on appetite suppression, it combines appetite regulation with effects on gastric emptying, making it a multifaceted approach to weight management.

3. Sustainability of Weight Loss:

The durability of the weight loss achieved with Ozempic is a notable factor. Unlike some fad diets or extreme weight loss measures that can result in quick but short-lived results, Ozempic promotes gradual, lasting weight loss, which is often easier to maintain over the long term.

4. Conditions comorbides :

Ozempic provides benefits to people with comorbidities, especially those with type 2 diabetes. The drug not only addresses weight concerns but also helps improve glycemic control and cardiovascular health, making it a comprehensive solution for people facing multiple health problems.

5. Comparison with bariatric surgery:

Although Ozempic does not replace bariatric surgery, it is a less invasive option for weight management. For people who may not be eligible or inclined for surgical procedures, Ozempic offers an alternative that can be integrated into their overall health plan.

6. Psychosocial Considerations:

The psychosocial aspects of weight loss are crucial. Ozempic's gradual approach may be more conducive to positive mental health, as it minimizes the risk of drastic changes that can impact body image and psychological well-being. This may be particularly relevant for people with a history of eating disorders or mental health issues.

7. Individual Preferences:

Weight loss methods are very individual and preferences play an important role in compliance. Some people may prefer the structured approach of medications like Ozempic, while others may thrive on personalized diet and exercise programs. The choice often depends on individual needs, preferences and recommendations of health care providers.

ADDRESSING CONCERNS ABOUT WEIGHT LOSS DURING TREATMENT

1. Monitoring weight changes:

Health care providers closely monitor weight changes during treatment with Ozempic. Regular check-ups, including assessments of weight, body composition and general health, allow for proactive adjustments to the treatment plan based on individual responses.

2. Individualized Treatment Plans:

Weight loss is not a unique result with Ozempic. Health care providers tailor treatment plans to individual needs, taking into account factors such as baseline weight, health status, and treatment goals. The goal is to achieve a healthy, sustainable weight that aligns with overall well-being.

3. Potential Concerns About Being Underweight:

Although weight loss is a common outcome, health care providers are vigilant about potential concerns related to being underweight or excessive weight loss. Monitoring nutritional status and addressing any signs of insufficient calorie intake are essential parts of comprehensive care.

4. Diet Tips:

Incorporating dietary advice into Ozempic treatment plans is common. Registered dietitians work with individuals to ensure their nutritional needs are met, particularly considering changes in appetite and eating habits associated with the use of Ozempic.

5. Focus on overall health:

Weight loss with Ozempic is considered in the broader context of overall health. The focus goes beyond the number on the scale to encompass improvements in metabolic health, cardiovascular risk factors and glycemic control.

6. Communication with healthcare providers:

Open and ongoing communication between individuals and their healthcare providers is crucial. Expressing concerns, discussing weight changes, and collaborating on treatment plan adjustments fosters a partnership that optimizes both diabetes management and weight-related outcomes.

7. Address psychological aspects:

The psychological aspects of weight loss, including issues with body image and emotional well-being, are addressed in health care. Incorporating mental health support, where necessary, ensures that the journey to a healthier weight is holistic and takes into account the individual's overall quality of life.

8. Incremental adjustments:

Healthcare providers are gradually approaching dosage adjustments of Ozempic, allowing individuals to adapt to changes in appetite and food intake. This gradual approach minimizes the risk of rapid and extreme weight loss, promoting a more balanced and lasting result.

CHAPTER 10

OZEMPIC AND HEART HEALTH

The relationship between diabetes, heart disease and stroke Diabetes, particularly type 2 diabetes, is closely linked to cardiovascular complications, including heart disease and stroke. This complex relationship arises from the impact of diabetes on multiple physiological processes, such as insulin resistance, inflammation and oxidative stress. People with diabetes are often at higher risk of developing atherosclerosis, a disease in which plaque builds up in the arteries, leading to narrowing and hardening of blood vessels.

1. Insulin resistance and atherosclerosis:

Insulin resistance, characteristic of type 2 diabetes, contributes to the development of atherosclerosis. When cells become resistant to the effects of insulin, blood sugar levels rise, triggering inflammation and damage to blood vessel walls. This sets the stage for the buildup of fatty deposits, or plaque, which can ultimately lead to heart disease and stroke.

2. Inflammation and oxidative stress:

Chronic inflammation and oxidative stress further exacerbate cardiovascular risks in people with diabetes. Elevated levels of inflammatory markers and oxidative stress markers are associated with the progression of atherosclerosis and increased likelihood of adverse cardiovascular events.

3. Diabetes as a cardiovascular risk factor:

Diabetes is recognized as a major cardiovascular risk factor. People with diabetes are at significantly higher risk of developing coronary heart disease, heart failure, and having a stroke. This increased risk highlights the importance of considering cardiovascular health as an integral component of diabetes management.

HOW OZEMPIC CAN IMPROVE THE HEART HEALTH OF PEOPLE WITH DIABETES

Ozempic, a GLP-1 receptor agonist, has emerged not only as a powerful tool for managing blood sugar levels in people with type 2 diabetes, but also as a drug with potential cardiovascular benefits. The following sections explain how Ozempic can help improve the heart health of people with diabetes.

1. Impact on insulin sensitivity:

One of the main mechanisms by which Ozempic improves heart health is by improving insulin sensitivity. As a GLP-1 receptor agonist, Ozempic increases the body's response to insulin, promoting better glucose utilization. Improved insulin sensitivity reduces strain on the cardiovascular system by addressing a key driver of atherosclerosis.

2. Blood sugar control:

The main function of Ozempic is to regulate blood sugar levels by increasing insulin secretion and reducing glucagon release. This not only helps achieve and maintain optimal glycemic control, but also helps reduce cardiovascular risk. By preventing prolonged periods of hyperglycemia, Ozempic indirectly protects the cardiovascular system from the harmful effects of hyperglycemia.

3. Benefits of Weight Management:

Weight management is a crucial aspect of cardiovascular health, and combining Ozempic with weight loss adds another level of benefits. Excess weight is often linked to cardiovascular risk factors such as high blood pressure and abnormal lipid profiles. Ozempic's ability to induce weight loss may positively influence these risk factors, helping to improve heart health.

4. Regulation of blood pressure:

Ozempic has been shown to have hypotensive effects, a key factor in reducing the risk of heart disease and stroke. By improving blood vessel function and promoting vasodilation, Ozempic helps maintain optimal blood pressure levels.

5. Cardiovascular protection beyond glycemic control:

Beyond its effects on blood sugar, Ozempic has demonstrated cardiovascular protection that goes beyond what can be attributed solely to glycemic control. This suggests that the drug may have direct positive effects on the cardiovascular system, thereby reducing the risk of major adverse cardiovascular events (MACE) in people with type 2 diabetes.

6. Reduce inflammation and oxidative stress:

Inflammation and oxidative stress, key players in the progression of cardiovascular diseases, are modulated by Ozempic. Studies suggest that GLP-1 receptor agonists, including Ozempic, exhibit anti-inflammatory and antioxidant properties. These actions can help reduce the inflammatory load on blood vessels, thereby promoting a healthier cardiovascular environment.

RESEARCH STUDIES ON OZEMPIC AND CARDIOVASCULAR OUTCOMES

Scientific research into the cardiovascular consequences associated with the use of Ozempic has provided valuable information, shaping our understanding of the drug's impact on the heart health of people with diabetes.

1. SUSTAIN Tests:

The SUSTAIN clinical trial program, comprising multiple studies, was instrumental in evaluating the cardiovascular safety and effectiveness of Ozempic. Notably, the SUSTAIN-6 trial demonstrated a significant reduction in the risk of major adverse cardiovascular events (MACE), including cardiovascular death, non-fatal myocardial infarction, and non-fatal stroke, in people treated with Ozempic compared to a placebo.

2. PIONEER Trials:

The PIONEER clinical trial program, focused on the efficacy and safety of Ozempic in a broad spectrum of people with type 2 diabetes, also provided relevant cardiovascular information. Although these trials primarily evaluated glycemic control, they provided valuable data on cardiovascular outcomes, supporting the overall cardiovascular safety profile of Ozempic.

3. SELECT Trial:

The SELECT trial, designed to evaluate the impact of Ozempic on cardiovascular outcomes, reinforced the cardiovascular safety of the drug. This trial specifically focused on people with type 2 diabetes and established cardiovascular disease, providing crucial data for this high-risk population.

4. Essai DECLARE-TIMI 58:

The DECLARE-TIMI 58 trial, which included a large and diverse population of people with type 2 diabetes, further examined the cardiovascular safety of Ozempic. The trial demonstrated that Ozempic did not increase the risk of MACE and, notably, showed potential benefits in reducing the risk of cardiovascular death.

5. Effects on heart failure:

Beyond traditional cardiovascular endpoints, studies have explored the effects of Ozempic on heart failure. The PIONEER 6 trial, for example, demonstrated that Ozempic reduces the risk of heart failure in people with type 2 diabetes.

CHAPTER 11

OZEMPIC AND PREGNANCY

Managing diabetes during pregnancy presents a unique set of challenges and considerations. For people using Ozempic, a GLP-1 receptor agonist, concerns arise about the potential risks and benefits associated with its use during pregnancy. In this exploration, we will delve into the intricacies of Ozempic and pregnancy, discuss the risks and benefits, provide guidelines for its use during pregnancy, and explore alternative treatment options for pregnant women with diabetes.

RISKS AND BENEFITS OF USING OZEMPIC DURING PREGNANCY

1. Potential risks:

The use of medications during pregnancy requires careful evaluation, and Ozempic is no exception. Limited data are available on the safety of Ozempic particularly during pregnancy, and the potential risks to the developing fetus are not fully understood. As a precaution, health care providers often use caution when considering the use of Ozempic in pregnant people.

2. Placental transfer:

Although Ozempic is a large molecule that is not expected to cross the placenta easily, there are concerns about its potential effects on the developing fetus. The limited studies available on the placental transfer of Ozempic suggest that it is unlikely to reach the developing fetus in significant quantities, but further research is needed to confirm these findings.

3. Lack of human studies:

Currently, there are few human studies specifically investigating the safety of Ozempic during pregnancy. Most data come from animal studies and extrapolation of these results to humans requires caution due to interspecies differences in drug metabolism and placental transfer.

4. Maternal weight loss:

Ozempic is associated with weight loss, which may be an unintended consequence during pregnancy. Weight loss during pregnancy, especially if it is excessive, can pose risks to both the mother and the developing fetus. Maintaining appropriate weight gain is crucial for a healthy pregnancy, and the potential impact of Ozempic-induced weight loss requires careful consideration.

5. Glycemic control and fetal development:

On the positive side, maintaining optimal glycemic control during pregnancy is essential to prevent complications such as birth defects, macrosomia (excess birth weight), and neonatal hypoglycemia. If Ozempic can contribute to effective blood sugar management without compromising fetal development, it could provide benefits by mitigating some of the risks associated with uncontrolled diabetes during pregnancy.

GUIDELINES FOR USE OF OZEMPIC DURING PREGNANCY

1. Individualized risk-benefit assessment:

The decision to use Ozempic during pregnancy should be based on an individualized risk/benefit assessment. Health care providers weigh the potential risks of exposure to Ozempic against the benefits of maintaining optimal blood sugar control during pregnancy. This assessment takes into account factors such as the severity of diabetes, pre-existing maternal conditions, and the overall health of the mother and fetus.

2. Preconception planning:

Ideally, discussions about the use of medications, including Ozempic, should take place during preconception planning. This allows healthcare providers to work with individuals to optimize blood sugar control before conception, thereby reducing the risks associated with uncontrolled diabetes during the early stages of pregnancy.

3. Patient Education:

Patient education is a crucial part of the decision-making process. Individuals should be informed of the limited data available on the use of Ozempic during pregnancy, the potential risks, and the importance of maintaining glycemic control. Open and transparent dialogue between healthcare providers and individuals ensures that informed decisions are made collaboratively.

4. Monitoring and adjustments:

If Ozempic is continued during pregnancy, close monitoring of maternal and fetal well-being is essential. Regular check-ups, including assessments of blood sugar, maternal weight and fetal development, allow timely adjustment of the treatment plan if necessary. This proactive approach helps optimize outcomes for the mother and fetus.

5. Consideration of alternative medications:

In some cases, healthcare providers may explore alternative medications with a more established safety profile during pregnancy. Insulin, for example, remains a mainstay of diabetes management during pregnancy and is often considered a safer option when there is uncertainty about using newer medications like Ozempic.

6. Multidisciplinary approach:

Management of diabetes in pregnancy is a collaborative effort that often involves a multidisciplinary team including obstetricians, endocrinologists, and maternal-fetal medicine specialists. This team approach ensures that decisions regarding medication use are well informed and take into account the unique aspects of pregnancy.

ALTERNATIVE TREATMENT OPTIONS FOR PREGNANT WOMEN WITH DIABETES

1. Insulin therapy:

Insulin remains the gold standard for diabetes management during pregnancy. It has been used for a long time and its safety profile is well established. Insulin can effectively control blood sugar levels while minimizing potential risks to the developing fetus.

2. Oral medications:

Some oral medications, such as metformin and glyburide, have been used in some cases during pregnancy. However, their safety profiles are better established and they are often considered when insulin alone does not provide adequate blood sugar control.

3. Continuous Glucose Monitoring (CGM):

Continuous glucose monitoring (CGM) has become an integral part of diabetes management during pregnancy. CGM allows real-time monitoring of blood sugar levels, providing valuable data to make informed adjustments to insulin therapy or other interventions.

4. Lifestyle Changes:

Lifestyle modifications, including dietary changes and regular exercise, play a crucial role in managing diabetes during pregnancy. Working with dietitians and healthcare providers to create a tailored meal plan and exercise routine can help with blood sugar control.

5. Regular Antenatal Care:

Regular prenatal care is essential to monitor the health of the mother and fetus. Prenatal appointments allow healthcare providers to assess maternal blood sugar levels, monitor fetal development, and respond quickly to any emerging concerns.

6. Reduction of risk factors:

It is important to manage other risk factors that may contribute to complications during pregnancy. This involves addressing factors such as hypertension, hyperlipidemia and lifestyle habits that can impact maternal and fetal health.

Made in the USA
Middletown, DE
09 February 2024

49378139R00073